Copycat] for Beginners

New and updated recipes from famous restaurants to enjoy a lot of amazing and appetizing dishes.
Start cooking like in the most exclusive restaurant in town.

JORDAN BERGSTROM

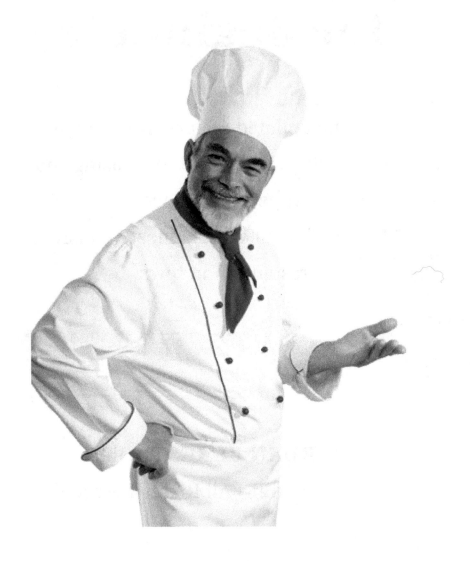

Table of Contents

PIZZA RECIPES..61

VEGAN RECIPES...86

INTRODUCTION

It is now easy to prepare and enjoy recipes from your favorite restaurants at the comfort of your home, thanks to copycat recipes.

With copycat recipes, you get to save your money and have fun enjoying your favorite meals. You can make many different recipes from various famous restaurants around the world. It can be a dessert from Applebee or a steak from Texas Roadhouse that you have always been enjoying. It can also be from Cheesecake Factory, Olive Garden, McDonald's, or Starbucks. If you are a lover of the restaurants' great recipes, they are easy to make, and the processes are not complex.

Once you learn how to make the delicious recipes at your home, you will not need to visit the restaurants as often as you did before make copycat recipes. Copycat recipes are available online, and you can easily find the copycat recipes you want. Youkan read them at your leisure, and you can prepare the recipes at home. The best part of it all is that you do not have to pay for expensive recipes. With these copycat recipes, you can actually save a lot of money.

Copycat recipes are based on home-cooked food. In addition to making a recipe like that of any restaurant, you have the opportunity to make some modification of choice to the recipe you are making. They will give you positive changes in the way you prepare them. You will not want to turn back once you go the way of copycat recipes. There are high calories in food prepared in restaurants, and you also do not know the nutrition info of the food. While preparing copycat recipes at home, you get to make healthy meals which you can know the nutritional info.

Copycat recipe books are designed for people who love eating out at restaurants. They give you the same recipes as the ones you can get in restaurants. So, you do not have to spend money exiting your home to get your favorite meal from a restaurant. When you want to enjoy a meal and have fun, it is nice when you can make it in your own home.

These copycat recipe books will make your time at home more enjoyable. You can get any recipe you want from these books, and it is easy to prepare them. When you have the copycat recipe book, you can prepare a tasty meal in no time. They are fun to use as they give you an idea on how to make the healthy meals at your home.

The copycat recipe book will serve you best when you want to make a meal for your family. You can also use it when you want to entertain your friends at home. When they eat the food at your place, they will think that you are a great cook, and they will admire the kind of food you have served them. They will also appreciate what you have done for them.

BREAKFAST RECIPES

Low Carb Banana Bread (Starbucks)

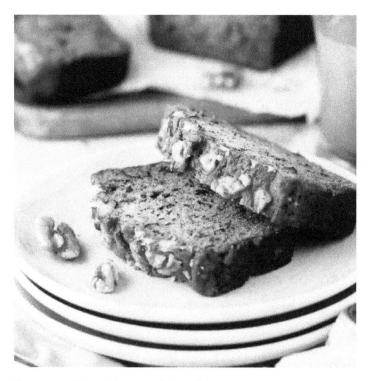

Preparation time: 11 minutes

Cooking time: 62 minutes

Servings: 6

Ingredients:

For dry ingredients:

- 2 tablespoons coconut flour
- 1 cup blanched almond flour

- ¼ cup chopped walnuts
- 1 teaspoon ground cinnamon
- 1 teaspoon baking powder
- 1/8 teaspoon salt (optional)
- ¼ teaspoon xanthan gum (optional)

For wet ingredients:

- ¼ cup allulose
- 2 large eggs
- 1 teaspoon banana extract
- 2 tablespoons unsweetened almond milk
- 3 tablespoons butter

Directions:

1. Prep small loaf pan (8 x 4 inches) with a large sheet of parchment paper so that it overhangs from it (on the width sides).
2. Stir in all the dry ingredients into a bowl and stir well.
3. Add allulose and butter to a bowl and mix with an electric mixer until creamy.
4. Whisk eggs and beat on low speed until well combined. Beat in the almond milk and banana extract.
5. Incorporate dry ingredients with the wet ingredients. Continue beating on low speed until smooth and free from lumps.

6. Add walnuts and stir.

7. Scoop the batter into the prepared loaf pan.

8. Bake at 350F for about 5 minutes or until brown on top.

9. Situate in the pan to cool completely. Lift the bread along with the parchment paper and carefully peel off the paper.

10.   Cut into 6 equal slices and serve. You should get slices of about 1 ¾ inch thick. The nutritional value mentioned is of this size.

Nutrition 224 Calories 20g Fat 8g Protein

Chicken Nuggets (McDonald's)

Preparation time: 10 minutes

Cooking time: 2 minutes

Servings: 10

Ingredients:

For chicken nuggets:

- 44.44 ounces boneless skinless chicken breasts, diced
- 2 eggs
- 2 teaspoons black pepper
- 2 teaspoons onion powder
- 2 teaspoons garlic powder
- 2 teaspoons paprika
- 3 teaspoons salt or to taste
- 2.12 ounces blanched almond flour (about ½ cup)
- 4 teaspoons parsley

For breading:

- ¾ cup egg white powder
- Oil to fry, as required + extra to grease your hands
- 4 eggs, beaten

Directions:

1. Place a deep fryer pan over medium flame. Pour enough oil in the pan and let the oil heat to 280 - 300º F.

2. Add all the ingredients for chicken nuggets into the food processor bowl. Blend until finely ground.

3. Line a baking sheet with parchment paper. Grease your hands with a little oil whenever required.

4. Divide the mixture into 80 equal portions and shape into nuggets. Keep them on the baking sheet. Use around a tablespoon of the chicken mixture for a nugget.

5. Place egg white powder in a shallow bowl.

6. Dip the chicken nuggets in egg, one at a time. You can pick up the nugget using a fork. Shaking off the extra egg, dredge the nugget in egg white powder and place it back on the baking sheet.

7. Carefully add 6 – 8 chicken nuggets in the hot oil. Cook until golden brown.

8. Pull out and put on a plate lined with paper towels.

9. Fry the remaining chicken pieces similarly.

Nutrition 222 Calories 8.6g Fat 35g Protein

Cheddar Bay Biscuits (Red Lobster)

Preparation time: 13 minutes

Cooking time: 12 minutes

Servings: 18

Ingredients:

- 3 cups superfine almond flour
- 2 tablespoons baking powder
- 4 large eggs
- 8 tablespoons unsalted butter, melted
- 1 cup sour cream
- 2 teaspoons garlic powder
- ½ teaspoon salt
- 1 cup grated cheddar cheese

For garlic butter topping:

- 4 tablespoons butter, melted
- 2 tablespoons minced parsley
- 1 teaspoon garlic powder

Directions:

1. Grease 3 muffin pans of 6 counts each with some cooking spray.
2. Add almond flour, garlic powder and baking powder into a bowl and mix well

3. Stir together sour cream, eggs and butter in a bowl. Transfer mixture into the bowl of dry ingredients. Stir until you get sticky dough.
4. Add cheese and stir.
5. Divide the batter into the muffin pans.
6. Bake in oven at 450F for 12 minutes.
7. Remove the muffin pans from the oven and allow it to cool for a few minutes. Slice around the edges to loosen the biscuits.
8. To make garlic butter topping: add butter, garlic powder and parsley into a small bowl and mix well.
9. Get the baking sheet out of the oven. Brush the biscuits with butter mixture and allow them to cool for a few minutes.
10.   Serve.

Nutrition 240 Calories 22g Fat 7g Protein

Chicken Bites with Sweet Mustard Dipping Sauce (Chick-Fil-A)

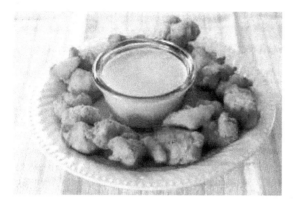

Preparation time: 81 minutes

Cooking time: 22 minutes

Servings: 8

Ingredients:

For mustard sauce:

- 1 cup mayonnaise
- 4 teaspoons apple cider vinegar
- ½ teaspoon turmeric powder
- 20 – 30 drops liquid stevia
- 4 teaspoons Dijon mustard
- 1 teaspoon garlic powder
- ½ teaspoon onion powder

For chicken:

- 2 pounds hand-trimmed chicken breast, cut into 1-inch pieces

- 1 teaspoon coarse kosher salt
- 2 tablespoons baking powder
- 2 teaspoons salt or to taste
- 1 teaspoon paprika
- Oil to fry, as required
- 3 tablespoons pickle juice
- 1 cup unflavored whey protein isolate
- 2 tablespoons erythritol
- 1 teaspoon garlic powder
- 1 teaspoon pepper

Directions:

1. To make mustard sauce: add all the ingredients for the mustard sauce into an airtight container and stir until well incorporated.
2. Cover the lid and refrigerate until use. It can last for 15 days.
3. To make chicken: add pickle juice and kosher salt into a large Ziploc bag. Seal the bag and shake until mix.
4. Add chicken and seal the bag. Shake the bag well. Chill for at least an hour. Flip the bag around a couple of times during this time.
5. Take out the bag from the refrigerator 30 minutes before frying.

6. Place a deep fryer pan over medium flame. Pour enough oil in the pan and let the oil heat to 350º F.

7. Meanwhile, add whey protein powder, erythritol, garlic powder, pepper, baking powder, salt and paprika into a shallow bowl and stir well.

8. Dredge chicken pieces in the mixture, one at a time and place on a lined baking sheet.

9. Carefully add a few of the chicken bites in the hot oil. Turn the bites so that they are golden brown on all sides.

10. Pull out and situate on a plate lined with paper towels.

11. Fry the remaining bites similarly.

12. Serve chicken bites with mustard sauce.

Nutrition 284 Calories 17g Fat 34g Protein

Chicken Strips (KFC)

Preparation time: 8 minutes

Cooking time: 7 minutes

Servings: 6

Ingredients:

- 2 chicken thighs, boneless, cut each into 3 pieces
- 1 ½ teaspoon KFC seasoning or to taste
- Oil to fry, as required
- ¾ cup almond flour
- 1 egg, beaten

Directions:

1. Place a deep fryer pan over medium flame. Pour enough oil in the pan and let the oil heat to 350° F.
2. Meanwhile, add almond flour and KFC seasoning to a shallow bowl and stir well.
3. Dredge chicken pieces in the almond flour mixture, one at a time.
4. Next dip the chicken pieces in egg, shaking off the extra egg, dredge once again in the almond flour mixture then situate on a lined baking sheet.
5. Carefully add 2 – 3 of the chicken pieces in the hot oil. Cook until golden brown.
6. Remove chicken strips and place on a plate.

7. Fry the remaining chicken pieces similarly.

Nutrition 218 Calories 17g Fat 8g Protein

Lasagna Dip (Olive Garden)

Preparation time: 11 minutes

Cooking time: 32 minutes

Servings: 5

Ingredients:

- ½ pound ground beef or turkey
- 1 cup unsalted canned, crushed tomatoes
- ¾ teaspoon minced garlic
- ¾ cup fat-free cottage cheese or ricotta cheese
- ½ tablespoon olive oil
- 2 tablespoons tomato paste
- 2 tablespoons minced red onion
- ¾ cup shredded, low-fat mozzarella cheese

Directions:

1. Place a skillet over medium flame. Pour the oil and allow it to heat. Add beef and cook until it turns brown.
2. Add tomatoes, garlic, tomato paste and onion and mix well.
3. Lower the heat and cook for 5 – 6 minutes. Turn off the heat.
4. Spread cottage cheese on the bottom of a baking dish. Spread the meat mixture over it.
5. Sprinkle mozzarella cheese.

6. Bake at 350F for 12 minutes.

Nutrition 160 Calories 6g Fat 19g Protein

Queso Blanco (Applebee's)

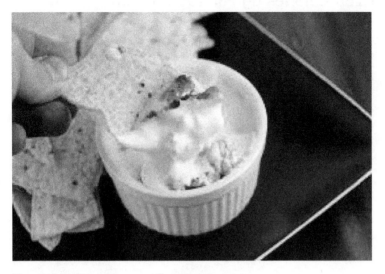

Preparation time: 6 minutes

Cooking time: 14 minutes

Servings: 20

Ingredients:

- 4 tablespoons vegetable oil
- 2/3 cup finely chopped white onion
- 16 ounces Monterey Jack cheese, chopped into chunks
- 1 cup chopped tomato
- ¼ cup finely minced jalapeño pepper
- 2 pounds white American cheese, chopped into chunks
- 1 cup half and half
- ¼ cup chopped cilantro

Directions:

1. Place a pan with oil, over medium-low heat. Once the oil is heated, add most of the jalapeño pepper, onions and cook for 5 minutes.
2. Add both kinds of cheese and half and half and mix well. Reduce the heat and cook until the cheese melts.
3. Add the tomatoes and half the cilantro. Mix it well then cook for 2 minutes.
4. Sprinkle remaining jalapeño and cilantro on top and serve.

Nutrition 295 Calories 25g Fat 14g Protein

Cream Cheese Dip (Rotel)

Preparation time: 6 minutes

Cooking time: 13 minutes

Servings: 5

Ingredients:

- ½ pound ground sausage, hot or mild
- ½ container sour cream
- ½ package cream cheese, softened
- ½ package Velveeta cheese
- 1 ½ tablespoon diced jalapeño peppers
- 1 can Mexican Rotel tomatoes

Directions:

1. Place a saucepan over medium flame. Add sausage and cook until it turns brown. Turn off the heat. Discard the cooked fat.
2. Meanwhile, add cream cheese, sour cream and Velveeta into a microwave-safe bowl and cook on high for 90 seconds. Stir a couple of times while melting.
3. Transfer the sausage and melted mixture into a crockpot. Mix well and keep it warm.

Nutrition 251 Calories 18g Fat 12g Protein

Queso (Pappasito's)

Preparation time: 7 minutes

Cooking time: 11 minutes

Servings: 4

Ingredients:

- ¾ pound American cheese, shredded
- ½ tablespoon minced garlic
- 3 tablespoons whole milk
- 1/8 teaspoon garlic salt
- 2 ounces canned green chilies with its liquid
- ¼ cup finely chopped onion
- ¼ cup, deseeded, fresh tomatoes

Directions:

1. Place cheese in a saucepan. Add milk and place the saucepan over low heat.
2. Stir frequently until the mixture melts.
3. Stir in chilies, onion and garlic salt and cook for a few minutes until onions are slightly soft. Pour in more milk if the mixture is very thick.
4. Turn off the heat.
5. Stir in the tomatoes and serve.

Nutrition 327 Calories 27g Fat 15g Protein

MAIN RECIPES

Chicken and Dumplings

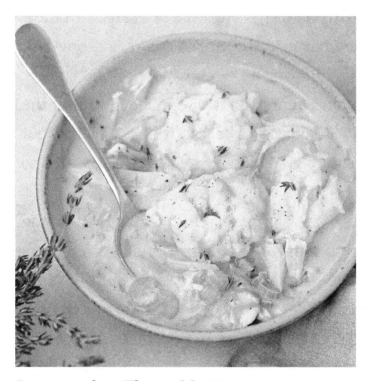

Preparation Time: 30 Minutes

Cooking Time: 20 Minutes

Servings: 4

Ingredients:

- 2 cups flour
- ½ teaspoon baking powder 1 pinch salt
- 2 tablespoons butter 1 scant cup buttermilk

- 2 quarts chicken broth
- 3 cups cooked chicken

Directions:

1. Make the dumplings by compounding the flour, baking powder and salt in a large bowl. By means of a pastry cutter or two knives, cut the butter into the flour mixture. Stir in the milk a tiny at a time until it forms a dough ball.
2. Cover your countertop with enough flour that the dough will not stick when you roll it out. Roll out the dough relatively thin, then cut into squares to form dumplings.
3. Flour a plate and transfer the dough from the counter to the plate.
4. Bring the chicken broth to a boil in a large saucepan, then drop the dumplings in one by one, stirring continually. The excess flour will thicken the broth.
5. Cook for about 20 minutes or pending the dumplings are no longer doughy.
6. Add the chicken, stir to combine, and serve.

Nutrition: Calories: 323 Fat: 78g Carbs: 87 g Protein: 69 g Sodium: 769 mg

Chicken Pot Pie

Preparation Time: 30 Minutes

Cooking Time: 30 Minutes

Servings: 8

Ingredients:

- ½ cup butter
- 1 medium onion, diced
- 1 (14.5-ounce) can chicken broth
- 1 cup half and half milk
- ½ cup all-purpose flour
- 1 carrot, diced
- 1 celery stalk, diced
- 3 medium potatoes, peeled and diced
- 3 cups cooked chicken, diced
- ½ cup frozen peas
- 1 teaspoon chicken seasoning
- ½ teaspoon salt
- ½ teaspoon ground pepper
- 1 single refrigerated pie crust
- 1 egg
- Water

Directions:

1. Preheat the oven to 375°F.

2. In a large frypan, heat the butter over medium heat, add the leeks and sauté for 3 minutes.

3. Sprinkle flour over the mixture, and remain to stir constantly for 3 minutes.

4. Whisking constantly, blend in the chicken broth and milk. Bring the mixture to a boil. Reduce heat to medium-low.

5. Add the carrots, celery, potatoes, salt, pepper, and stir to combine. Cook for 10-15 minutes or pending veggies are cooked through but still crisp. Add chicken and peas. Stir to combine.

6. Transfer chicken filling to a deep 9-inch pie dish.

7. Fit the pie crust sheet on top and press the edges around the dish to seal the crust. Trim the excess if needed.

8. In a distinct bowl, whisk an egg with 1 tablespoon of water, and brush the mixture over the top of the pie. With a knife, cut a few slits to let steam escape.

9. Bake the pie in the oven on the middle oven rack 20 to 30 minutes until the crust becomes golden brown.

10. Let the pie rest for about 15 minutes before serving.

Nutrition: Calories: 125 Fat: 43 g Carbs: 76 g Protein: 65 g Sodium: 545 mg

Chang's Mongolian Beef

Preparation Time: 10 Minutes

Cooking Time: 20 Minutes

Servings: 2

Ingredients:

- 1 pound flank steak
- ¼ cup cornstarch
- 2 teaspoons
- ½ teaspoon ginger, finely chopped
- 1 tablespoon ginger, diced
- ½ soy sauce
- ½ cup water
- ½ cup brown sugar
- 1 cup vegetable oil, divided
- 6 green onions, cut diagonally into 2-inch pieces

Directions:

1. Cut steak against the grain into small pieces, about ¼ inch. Transfer steak into a bowl with cornstarch and flip until fully coated on all sides. Set aside.

2. In a frypan, heat 1 tablespoon of the oil on medium heat. Stir in ginger and garlic. Cook for about 1 minute or pending aromatic. Mix in soy sauce, water, and brown sugar. Keep stirring until

sugar is melted. Bring to a boil on medium heat. Simmer for around 2 minutes or until sauce is thick.

3. Heat remaining vegetable oil in a separate saucepan on medium heat until oil reaches 350 F. Deep-fry steak in batches for 2 minutes or until brown.

4. Handover onto a plate lined with paper towels.

5. Discard the oil, then add sauce and stir in meat with sauce in saucepan for about 2 minutes on medium heat. Mix in green onions and cook for an

6. additional 1-2 minute. Place meat and onions on a plate.

7. Serve hot.

Nutrition: Calories: 847 Fat: 24 g Carbs: 103 g Protein: 57 g Sodium: 4176 mg

Sizzling Steak, Cheese, and Mushrooms Skillet from Applebee's

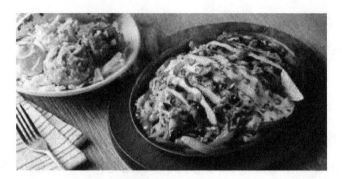

Preparation Time: 15 Minutes

Cooking Time: 1 Hour and 35 Minutes

Servings: 4

Ingredients:

- 1 head garlic, cut crosswise
- 2 tablespoons olive oil, divided
- Salt and pepper, to taste
- 2 pounds Yukon Gold potatoes,
- Water, for boiling
- 2 tablespoons butter
- 1 large yellow onion
- 8 ounces cremini mushrooms
- Salt and pepper to taste
- ½ cup milk
- ¼ cup cream
- 3 tablespoons butter

- 2½ pounds 1-inch-thick sirloin steak, cut into 4 large pieces
- 8 slices mozzarella cheese

Directions:

1. Preheat oven to 300°F.
2. Position garlic on foil. Pour 1 tablespoon olive oil to the inner sides where the garlic was cut, then wrap foil around garlic.
3. Put it in oven then bake for 30 minutes. Remove from oven, and squeeze out garlic from head. Transfer to a bowl or mortar. Add salt and pepper, then mash together. Set aside.
4. In a pot, add potatoes. Pour enough water on top to cover potatoes. Bring to a boil. Once boiling, reduce heat to medium. Simmer for about 20 to 25
5. minutes or until potatoes become tender.
6. Melt butter on a non-stick pan over medium-low heat. Add onions and sauté for about 15 minutes until a bit tender. Toss in mushrooms and sauté, adjusting heat to medium. Season with salt and pepper. Cook for 10 minutes more. Set aside and keep warm.
7. Drain potatoes, then mash using an electric mixer on low speed. While mashing, gradually pour in

milk, cream, butter, and mashed garlic with olive oil. Keep blending until everything is cream-like and smooth. Remove from mixer and place a cover on top of bowl. Set aside and keep warm.

8. Evenly coat steak pieces with remaining 1 tablespoon olive oil on all sides.

9. Heat grill, then place meat on grill. Cook for 4 minutes. Flip and add mozzarella slices on top. Cook for additional 4 minutes for medium rare. Add additional minutes for increased doneness.

10. Transfer steaks to serving plates then top with onion/mushroom mixture.

11. Place mashed potatoes on the side. Serve.

Nutrition: Calories: 1159 Fat: 60 g Saturated fat: 29 g Carbs: 47 g Sugar: 4 g Fibers: 6 g Protein: 107 g Sodium: 1495 mg

Panda Express' Beef and Broccoli

Preparation Time: 30 Minutes

Cooking Time: 15 Minutes

Servings: 4

Ingredients:

- 2 tablespoons cornstarch, divided
- 3 tablespoons Chinese rice wine, divided
- 1 pound flank steak, cut thinly against the grain
- 1 pound broccoli florets,
- 2 tablespoons oyster sauce
- 2 tablespoons water
- 1 tablespoon brown sugar
- 1 tablespoon soy sauce
- 1 tablespoon cornstarch
- 2 tablespoons canola oil
- ¼ teaspoon sesame oil
- 1 teaspoon ginger, finely chopped
- 2 cloves garlic, finely chopped
- 2 teaspoons sesame seeds

Directions:

1. In a big Ziploc bag, add 1 tablespoon cornstarch and 2 tablespoons Chinese rice wine. Place beef inside and seal tightly. Massage bag to fully coat beef.

41

2. Set aside to marinate for at minimum 20 minutes.

3. Rinse broccoli and place in a nonreactive bowl. Put a wet paper towel, then microwave for 2 minutes. Set aside.

4. Stir oyster sauce, water, 1 tablespoon Chinese rice wine, brown sugar, soy sauce, and remaining cornstarch in a bowl until well mixed. Set aside.

5. Heat wok over high heat. You want the wok to be very hot. Then, heat canola and sesame oil in wok and wait to become hot. Working in batches, add steak and cook over high heat for 1 minute. Flip, then cook other side for extra 1 minute. Transfer to a plate.

6. To the same wok, add garlic and ginger. Sauté for about 10 to 15 seconds then return beef to wok. Toss in heated broccoli. Slightly stir prepared sauce to make sure cornstarch is not settled on the bottom, then add to wok. Toss everything in sauce to combine. Continue cooking until sauce becomes thick.

7. Garnish with sesame seeds. Serve.

Nutrition: Calories: 324 Fat: 17 g Saturated fat: 4g Carbs: 13 g Sugar: 6g Fibers: 3 g Protein: 28 g Sodium: 464 mg

Edo Japan's Sukiyaki Beef

Preparation Time: 15 Minutes

Cooking Time: 5 to 6 Minutes

Servings: 4

Ingredients:

- 10 ounces sirloin steak, thinly sliced
- ½ carrot, thinly sliced
- ½ onion, sliced
- 1 green pepper, sliced
- ½ yellow bell pepper, sliced
- ½ cup sukiyaki sauce, divided
- 1 tablespoon oil
- 1 teaspoon chopped garlic
- 2 tablespoons ginger, finely chopped
- 2 teaspoons soy sauce
- 1 teaspoon sugar
- 1 tablespoon oyster sauce

Directions:

1. Pour half of the sukiyaki sauce into a medium bowl and add the sliced beef.
2. Let the beef marinate for 20 minutes.
3. Heat the oil in a large skillet. Add the garlic and cook for about 30 seconds.

---

4. Add the beef, with the sauce. Cook over medium-high heat until the beef is cooked through.
5. Add the ginger, carrots, peppers and onions and cook until the veggies have begun to soften.
6. Add the rest of the sukiyaki sauce along with the oyster sauce, soy sauce and sugar. Cook and stir for around 2 more minutes.
7. Serve over rice.

Nutrition: Calories: 152 Fat: 24 g Carbs: 20 g Protein: 5.6 g Sodium: 627 mg

Broccoli Cheddar Chicken

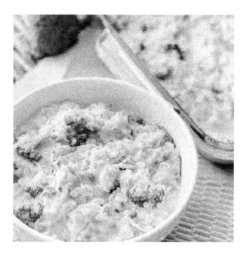

Preparation Time: 10 Minutes

Cooking Time: 45 Minutes

Servings: 4

Ingredients:

- 4 skinless chicken breasts
- 1 cup milk
- 1 cup Ritz-style crackers, crushed
- 1 can condensed cheddar cheese soup ½ pound frozen broccoli
- 6 ounces cheddar cheese, shredded
- ½ teaspoon salt
- ½ teaspoon pepper

Directions:

1. Preheat the oven to 350°F.

2. Whisk the milk and cheddar cheese soup together in a mixing bowl.

3. Prepare a baking dish by greasing the sides, then lay the chicken in the bottom and season with the salt and pepper.

4. Pour the soup combination over the chicken, then top with the crackers, broccoli and shredded cheese.

5. Bake for around 45 minutes or until bubbly.

Nutrition: Calories: 343 Fat: 43 g Carbs: 54 g Protein: 16 g Sodium: 565 mg

DRESSING AND SAUCE RECIPES

Olive Garden Artichoke-Spinach Dip

Preparation Time: 13 minutes

Cooking Time: 4 hours

Servings: 16

Ingredients:

- 1 (12-ounce) jar roasted sweet red peppers
- 1 (6½-ounce) jar marinated quartered artichoke hearts
- 1 (10-ounce) package frozen chopped spinach, thawed and squeezed dry
- 6 ounces cream cheese, softened and cubed
- 1½ cups Asiago cheese, shredded
- 8 ounces fresh mozzarella cheese, cubed
- 1 cup feta cheese, crumbled
- 1/3 cup provolone cheese, shredded
- 2 tablespoons mayonnaise
- 1/3 cup fresh basil, minced
- ¼ cup onion, chopped finely

- 2 garlic cloves, minced

Direction

1. Drain the jar of roasted peppers, reserving 1 tablespoon of liquid.
2. Then, chop the peppers.
3. Drain the jar of artichokes, reserving 2 tablespoons of liquid.
4. Then, chop the artichokes roughly.
5. In a greased slow cooker, place all ingredients and stir to combine.
6. Add the reserved pepper and artichoke liquids and stir to combine.
7. Set the slow cooker on High and cook, covered for about 2 hours.
8. Uncover the slow cooker and stir the dip.
9. Set the slow cooker on High and cook, covered for about 30-60 minutes.
10. Uncover the slow cooker and stir the dip well.
11. Serve hot.

Nutrition 182 Calories 11g Proteins 13g Fat

Dean's French Onion Dip

Preparation Time: 14 minutes

Cooking Time: 37 minutes

Servings: 8

Ingredients:

- 2 tablespoons olive oil
- 2 large onions, chopped finely
- ¾ cup sour cream
- ¾ cup plain Greek yogurt
- 3 teaspoons onion powder
- ½ teaspoon salt

Direction

1. In a large skillet, heat the oil over medium heat and sauté the onions for about 5 minutes.
2. Reduce the heat to medium-low and cook for about 30 minutes, stirring occasionally.
3. Remove from the heat and set aside to cool completely.
4. In a small bowl, add the sour cream, yogurt, onion powder, and salt and mix well.
5. Add 2/3 of cooked onion and stir to combine.
6. Transfer the dip into a serving bowl and serve with the ping of remaining onions.

Nutrition 107 Calories 2g Proteins 8g Fat

Chimichurri Sauce

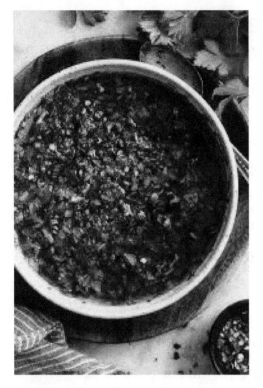

Preparation Time: 21 minutes

Cooking Time: 8 minutes

Servings: 4

Ingredients:

- 8 garlic cloves, minced
- Salt, as required
- 1 teaspoon dried oregano
- 1 teaspoon ground black pepper
- 1 teaspoon red pepper flakes, crushed
- 4-5 teaspoons lemon zest, grated finely

- 4 ounces fresh lemon juice
- 1 bunch fresh flat-leaf parsley
- 1 cup olive oil

Direction

1. For Chimichurri sauce: in a food processor, add all ingredients and pulse until well combined.

Nutrition 57 Calories 2g Proteins 5g Fat

Cheesecake Factory Cobb Salad Dressing

Preparation Time: 17 minutes

Cooking Time: 0 minutes

Servings: 6

Ingredients:

- 1 cup olive oil
- ¼ cup balsamic vinegar
- 1 teaspoon fresh lemon juice
- ¾ teaspoon Worcestershire sauce
- 1 small garlic clove, minced
- ¼ teaspoon Erythritol
- ¼ teaspoon ground mustard
- Salt and ground black pepper, as required

Direction

1. For dressing: in a blender, add all ingredients and pulse until smooth.
2. Transfer the dressing into a bowl and refrigerate before serving.

Nutrition 541 Calories 29g Proteins 46g Fat

Panera Bread Strawberry Salad Dressing

Preparation Time: 17 minutes

Cooking Time: 9 minutes

Servings: 8

Ingredients:

- ¼ cup homemade mayonnaise
- 1 tablespoon sour cream
- 1 tablespoon unsweetened almond milk
- 1 tablespoon Erythritol
- 2¼ teaspoons cider vinegar
- 1½ teaspoons poppy seeds

Direction

1. In a bowl, add all the ingredients and beat until well combined.
2. Place the dressing over salad and toss to coat well.

Nutrition 91 Calories 1.4g Proteins 7.7g Fat

McDonald's Big Mac Salad Dressing

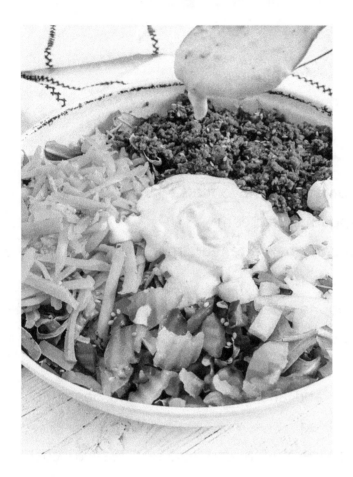

Preparation Time: 17 minutes

Cooking Time: 13 minutes

Servings: 4

Ingredients:

- ¾ cup homemade mayonnaise
- 2 tablespoons dill pickles
- 1 tablespoon onions, chopped

- 4 teaspoons prepared mustard
- 1 tablespoon balsamic vinegar
- 2 teaspoons Erythritol
- ½ teaspoon smoked paprika

Direction

1. For dressing: in a bowl, add all ingredients and mix well.

Nutrition 626 Calories 43g Proteins 48g Fat

The Cheesecake Factory's Tuna Tataki Salad Dressing

Preparation Time: 10 minutes

Cooking Time: 5 minutes

Servings: 4

Ingredients:

- 2 1-inch pieces of ginger, grated
- 2 tablespoons liquid stevia
- 4 tablespoons ponzu sauce, low-carb
- 2 tablespoons sake
- 2 tablespoons soy sauce
- 2 tablespoons toasted sesame oil

Directions:

1. Get a mason jar, place all of its ingredients in it, shut with the lid, and then shake well until well blended, set aside until required.

Nutrition: 594 Calories 42g Fats 37g Protein

Angry Alfredo Sauce from Olive Garden

Preparation Time: 10 minutes

Cooking Time: 25 minutes

Servings: 4

Ingredients:

For the Sauce:

- ½ cup of parmesan cheese – freshly grated
- 4 oz. of butter
- ½ tsp. garlic powder
- 1 cup of heavy cream
- ¼ tsp. red pepper chili flakes

Directions:

1. Warm a saucepan using the med-high heat setting to melt the butter. Be careful that the butter does not turn brown. Add the heavy cream, and wait till bubbles are formed. When bubbles begin to appear, add the cheese. Stir the ingredients frequently to ensure the sauce thickens to create a smooth consistency. Adjust the temperature to simmer on the stovetop. Add in the garlic powder and crushed pepper to the sauce.

Nutrition: 596 Calories 21g Protein 56g Fat

Chipotle Guacamole Sauce

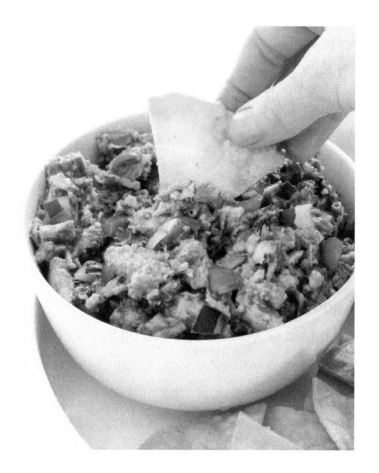

Preparation Time: 3 minutes

Cooking Time: 15 minutes

Servings: 2

Ingredients:

- 2 ripe avocados
- 1 lime
- ¼ cup red onion

- 6 grape tomatoes
- 1 clove of garlic
- 1 tbsp. olive oil
- 1/8 tsp. black pepper
- ¼ tsp. salt
- Fresh cilantro
- Optional: 1/8 tsp. crushed red pepper

Directions:

1. Do the prep. Juice the lime. Slice, remove the pit, and mash the avocados in a mixing container.
2. Dice the tomatoes and red onions. Add them to the avocado.
3. Mince the garlic clove and add the oil to combine.
4. Stir in the cilantro with the salt, pepper, crushed red pepper, and lime juice.
5. Thoroughly mix and serve with a steak bowl and a portion of pork rinds or low-carb crackers.

Nutrition: 155 Calories 2g Protein 14g Fat

PIZZA RECIPES

BBQ Chicken Pizza

Preparation time: 9 minutes

Cooking time: 39 minutes

Servings: 4

Ingredients

- Cooking spray
- 1 lb. refrigerated pizza dough, divided into 2 pieces
- 2 c. cooked shredded chicken
- 3/4 c. barbecue sauce, divided
- 1 c. shredded mozzarella
- 1/4 medium red onion, thinly sliced
- 1/3 c. shredded gouda
- Pinch crushed red pepper flakes (optional)
- 2 tbsp. freshly chopped cilantro

Directions

1. Preheat broiler to 500°. Line two huge preparing sheets with material paper and oil with cooking shower. In a medium bowl, mix together chicken and 1/4 cup grill sauce.

2. On a softly floured surface, turn out pizza batter into a huge circle, at that point slide onto the arranged heating sheet.

3. Top every pizza with 1/4 cup grill sauce, at that point a large portion of the chicken blend, spreading in an even layer and leaving 1" around the edge uncovered.

4. Next include an even layer of mozzarella and red onion, at that point top with gouda. Sprinkle with squashed red pepper pieces if utilizing. Prepare until cheddar is melty and the batter is cooked through 20 to 25 minutes. Trimming with cilantro before serving

Nutrition 499 calories 21g fat 14g protein

Pizza Pot Pie

Preparation time: 12 minutes

Cooking time: 38 minutes

Servings: 6

Ingredients

- 2 tbsp. extra-virgin olive oil, plus more for the crust
- 2 c. broccoli florets, roughly chopped
- 2 bell peppers, diced
- 8 oz. sliced mushrooms
- 1 lb. Italian sausage (sweet or spicy), casings removed
- 1/4 c. all-purpose flour, plus more for rolling dough
- 2 cloves garlic, minced
- 1 tsp. dried oregano
- Kosher salt
- Freshly ground black pepper 2 c.
- pizza sauce 1/2 lb.
- Refrigerated pizza dough 2 c
- shredded mozzarella 1/4 c.
- sliced pepperoni
- Freshly grated parmesan, for garnish
- Freshly chopped parsley, for garnish]

Directions

1. Preheat stove to 400°. In a 10-or 12-inch broiler-safe skillet over medium warmth, heat oil. Include broccoli and ringer peppers and cook, regularly mixing, until somewhat delicate, 5 minutes. Include mushrooms and cook, mixing, until delicate, 4 minutes more.

2. Include hotdog and cook, separating it with a wooden spoon, until burned and not, at this point pink, around 4 minutes.

3. Include flour and mix until vegetables and hotdog are very much covered, at that point include garlic and oregano and then season it with pepper and salt. Mix in pizza sauce and expel from heat. Let cool 10 minutes.

4. On a delicately floured surface, turn out pizza mixture into an enormous circle two or three inches greater than your skillet. Top frankfurter blend with mozzarella, at that point place batter round over skillet and cautiously crease edges.

5. Brush with oil and top with pepperoni. Heat until the covering is brilliant, around 40 minutes. Let cool 10 minutes, at that point sprinkle with parmesan and parsley before serving

Nutrition 391 calories 27g fat 19g protein

Primavera Skillet Pizza

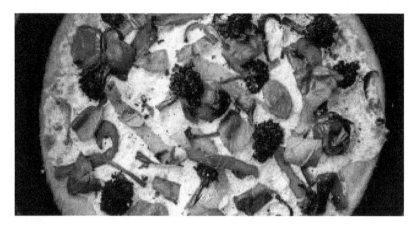

Preparation time: 13 minutes

Cooking time: 37 minutes

Servings: 4

Ingredients

- 2 bell peppers, sliced
- 1/2 head broccoli, florets removed
- 1/4 small red onion, thinly sliced
- 1 c. cherry tomatoes
- extra-virgin olive oil
- kosher salt
- Freshly ground black pepper
- All-purpose flour, for dusting surface
- 1 lb. pizza dough, at room temperature
- 1 c. ricotta
- 1 c. shredded mozzarella

Directions

1. Warmth broiler to 400°. On a huge heating sheet, hurl peppers, broccoli, onion, and cherry tomatoes with olive oil and season with salt and pepper. Cook until delicate and tomatoes are blasting, 18 to 20 minutes. Expel and increment broiler temperature to 500°.

2. In the meantime, brush a stove confirmation skillet with olive oil. On a floured work surface, utilize your hands to turn out the mixture until it's the periphery of your skillet. Move to skillet and brush mixture done with olive oil. Leaving a 1/2" fringe for covering, bit spoonful of ricotta on the batter and sprinkle with mozzarella. Top with simmered vegetables and sprinkle with olive oil. Sprinkle covering with salt. Heat until the covering is fresh and cheddar is dissolved around 12 minutes

Nutrition 391 calories 27g fat 22g protein

Bacon Weave Pizza

Preparation time: 14 minutes

Cooking time: 42 minutes

Servings: 4

Ingredients

- 12 slices thick-cut bacon
- 1/2 c. pizza sauce
- 1 c. shredded mozzarella
- 1 c. sliced green bell pepper
- 1/4 medium red onion, sliced
- 1/4 c. sliced black olives
- 1/4 c. grated parmesan

Directions

1. Preheat stove to 400°. Line an enormous heating sheet container with material paper.
2. To shape a bacon weave, line six bacon cuts one next to the other on the heating sheet.
3. Lift up and overlay back each other bacon cut, at that point lay the seventh cut on top in the middle.
4. Lay collapsed back cuts on the seventh cut, at that point crease back the substitute cuts. Spot eighth cut on top, close to the seventh cut, weaving as you did previously. Rehash this

procedure four additional occasions to finish the weave.

5. Spot a modified, broiler evidence cooling rack on the bacon cuts. This encourages them to remain level. Prepare 23 to 25 minutes, or until bacon begins too fresh.

6. Expel preparing sheet from the stove and pour off as much fat as possible. Cautiously expel rack, at that point spread with pizza sauce leaving ½-inch or so for the outside layer. Top with mozzarella, pepper, onions, olives, and parmesan.

7. Return sheet to broiler and keep heating until cheddar is melty, an additional 10 minutes.

Nutrition 391 calories 29g fat 17g protein

Bacon Pickle Pizza

Preparation time: 14 minutes

Cooking time: 32 minutes

Servings: 4

Ingredients

- 2 tbsp. extra-virgin olive oil
- 1 tsp. garlic powder
- 1 tsp. Italian seasoning
- premade pizza crust
- 1 1/2 c. mozzarella
- 1/4 c. freshly grated Parmesan
- 3/4 c. dill pickle slices
- 4 slices bacon, cooked and chopped
- 1 tbsp. freshly chopped dill
- 1/2 tsp. crushed red pepper flakes
- Ranch dressing, for serving, optional

Direction

1. Preheat broiler to 375° and fix an enormous heating sheet with material paper. Take a medium bowl, whisk together oil, Italian, and garlic powder flavoring—spot pizza hull on the arranged heating sheet and brush done with the oil blend.

2. Top hull with mozzarella and parmesan and heat until cheddar is melty, 15 minutes. Top with pickles and bacon and prepare 5 minutes more.
3. Top with dill and red pepper chips before presenting with the farm, if utilizing.

Nutrition 410 calories 31g fat 17g protein

BBQ Chicken Skillet Pizza

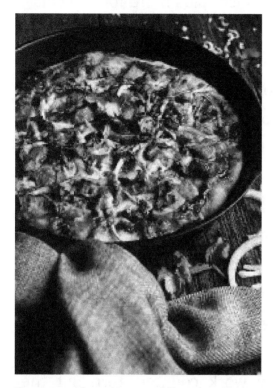

Preparation time: 12 minutes

Cooking time: 48 minutes

Servings: 4

Ingredients

- 1-tbsp. of extra-virgin olive oil
- ½-lb. of boneless skinless (cut into 1" pieces) chicken breasts
- Kosher salt
- Black pepper, grounded
- All-purpose flour, for dough 1 lb.

- pizza dough, at room temperature
- 2 tbsp. barbecue sauce, plus more for drizzling
- 1/2 c. shredded cheddar
- 1/2 c. shredded fontina
- 1/4 small red onion, thinly sliced
- Ranch dressing, for drizzling
- Freshly chopped chives, for garnish

Direction

1. Preheat stove to 500°. In an enormous skillet over medium-high warmth, heat oil. Include chicken and cook until brilliant and not, at this point pink, 6 minutes for every side—season liberally with salt and pepper.

2. In the meantime, brush an ovenproof skillet with oil. On a floured work counter, turn out the mixture until boundary coordinates your skillet. Move to skillet.

3. Leaving a 1/2" fringe for outside, spread grill sauce onto the batter. Top with cheddar, fontina, chicken, and red onion.

4. Brush covering with olive oil and sprinkle with salt. Heat until the outside is firm and cheddar is melty, 23 to 25 minutes.

5. Sprinkle with grill sauce and farm and embellishment with chives

Nutrition 399 calories 27g fats 14g protein

Zucchini Pizza Crust

Preparation time: 8 minutes

Cooking time: 39 minutes

Servings: 4

Ingredients

- 3-medium zucchini
- large egg
- cloves garlic, minced
- 1/2 tsp. Dried oregano
- c. shredded mozzarella, divided
- 1/2 c. grated Parmesan
- 1/4 c. cornstarch
- kosher salt Freshly ground black pepper
- 1/4 c. pizza sauce
- 1/4 c. pepperoni
- Pinch red pepper flakes, for garnish
- Basil, for garnish

Direction

1. Preheat stove to 425º and fix a preparing sheet with the material. On a case grater or in a food processor, grind zucchini. Utilizing cheesecloth or a drying towel, wring overabundance dampness out of zucchini.

2. Move zucchini to an enormous bowl with the egg, garlic, oregano, 1 cup mozzarella, parmesan, and cornstarch and season with salt and pepper. Mix until totally consolidated.
3. Move "mixture" to arranged preparing sheet and pat into an outside layer. Heat until brilliant and dried out 25 minutes.
4. Spread pizza sauce over an outside layer at that point top with outstanding mozzarella and pepperoni.
5. Prepare until cheddar is liquefied and the covering is fresh, around 10 minutes more—enhancement with red pepper pieces and basil.

Nutrition 497 calories 28g fat 15g protein

Slow-Cooker Pizza

Preparation time: 9 minutes

Cooking time: 42 minutes

Servings: 4

Ingredients

- Cooking spray, for slow cooker
- 1 lb. pizza dough
- 1 c. pizza sauce
- 2 c. shredded mozzarella
- 1/2 c. freshly grated Parmesan
- 1/2 c. sliced pepperoni
- 1/2 tsp. Italian seasoning
- pinch of crushed red pepper flakes
- 1 tsp. Freshly chopped parsley, for garnish

Direction

1. Splash base and sides of an enormous moderate cooker with nonstick cooking shower.
2. Press pizza batter into the base of moderate cooker until it arrives at all edges and base is totally secured.
3. Spoon over pizza sauce and spread, leaving around 1" of batter around edges. Top with cheeses, pepperoni, and flavors. Spread

moderate cooker and cook on low until outside turns brilliant and cheddar is melty, 3 to 4 hours.

4. Expel top and let cool 5 minutes. Utilizing a spatula, expel pizza from the simmering pot. Topping with parsley, at that point cut and serve.

Nutrition 391 calories 27g fat 14g protein

Grilled Pizza Bread

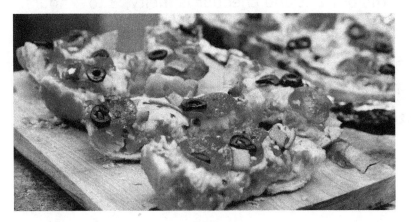

Preparation time: 13 minutes

Cooking time: 39 minutes

Servings: 4

Ingredients

- large loaf halved
- 15-oz. jar pizza sauce
- 2-c. of shredded mozzarella
- 1/3-c. of pepperoni
- 1/4-c. of black olives
- ½-red onion
- Green Bell Pepper, chopped
- pinch of crushed red pepper flakes

Direction

1. Scoop out the middles from both bread parts to make shallow vessels.

2. Spread pizza sauce onto every half at that point top with mozzarella, pepperoni, dark olives, red onion, green ringer pepper, and red pepper pieces.

3. Wrap bread freely with aluminum foil and spot over open-air fire (or on a hot flame broil) and cook until the cheddar is melty and the hull is toasted, 10 to 15 minutes.

4. Let cool for around 10 minutes until cutting.

Nutrition 391 calories 31g fat 19g protein

Toaster Pizza Tots

Preparation time: 14 minutes

Cooking time: 29 minutes

Servings: 4

Ingredients

- frozen monster tot (aka hash brown patty)
- 1 tbsp. pizza sauce
- tbsp. shredded mozzarella cheese
- 7 pepperoni slices (or to taste)
- Dried oregano, for garnish
- Red pepper flakes, for garnish (optional)

Direction

1. Set the toaster broiler to 400° and fix the plate with aluminum foil.
2. Put the tot on the plate and cook to brown on both sides, around 10 minutes. (Contingent upon your toaster stove, you may need to flip it or leave it in for various rounds. It is imperative to get it extremely firm before fixing it.)
3. Expel the tot from the toaster. Top with the sauce, at that point the cheddar, and afterward the pepperoni.
4. Return the tot to the toaster and toast again until the cheddar has dissolved and is beginning to

brown. Sprinkle with oregano and red pepper chips to taste. Serve hot.

Nutrition 419 calories 31g fat 24g protein

Low-Carb Breakfast Pizza

Preparation time: 14 minutes

Cooking time: 32 minutes

Servings: 4

Ingredients

- 4-large eggs
- 2 ½-c. of shredded mozzarella
- ¼-grated Parmesan
- kosher salt
- ¼-tsp. of Freshly ground black pepper.
- dried oregano
- pinch red pepper flakes
- 2-tbsp. pizza sauce
- ¼-c. mini pepperoni
- ½- chopped Green Bell Pepper

Direction

1. Preheat stove to 400° and fix a preparing sheet with material paper. In a medium bowl, join eggs, 2 cups mozzarella, and parmesan.

2. Mix until joined, at that point season with salt, pepper, oregano and red pepper drops. Spread blend into a ½" thick round on heating sheet.

3. Prepare until gently brilliant, around 12 minutes—spread pizza sauce on the heated hull.

4. Top with outstanding mozzarella, pepperoni, and chime pepper. Heat until cheddar is softened and outside layer is fresh, around 10 minutes more. Sprinkle with parmesan, if utilizing, before serving.

Nutrition 311 calories 22g fat 19g protein

Egg-in-a-Hole Pizza Bagels

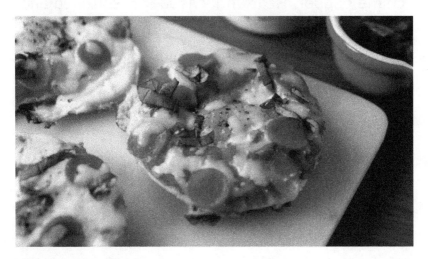

Preparation time: 8 minutes

Cooking time: 36 minutes

Servings: 4

Ingredients

- 2 tbsp. butter, divided
- 2 bagels, halved
- 1/2 c. pizza sauce
- 2 c. shredded mozzarella
- 1/3 c. mini pepperoni
- 2 tbsp. chopped fresh parsley
- 4 large eggs
- kosher salt
- Freshly ground black pepper
- Fresh basil, for garnish

Direction

1. Dissolve 1 tablespoon margarine in a nonstick skillet over medium warmth. At the point when the margarine has liquefied, place the bagel parts in the skillet chop sides down. Toast until brilliant.
2. Mood killer the warmth and spot the bagel parts on a plate, toasted sides up. Utilize a cutout (or little glass) to cut a greater gap in the focal point of the bagel and spread with pizza sauce and top with mozzarella and little pepperoni.
3. Wipe the skillet with a paper towel. Liquefy remaining spread over medium warmth and return the bagel to the skillet, pizza-side up. Break an egg in the focal point of each gap and season the egg with salt and pepper to taste.
4. Spread the skillet with an enormous top and cook until the cheddar has softened and the egg has arrived at wanted doneness, around 4 minutes for a runny just right egg.
5. Garnish with basil.

Nutrition 391 calories 31g fat 27g protein

VEGAN RECIPES

Applebee® Vegetable Medley

Preparation Time: 15 Minutes

Cooking Time: 10 Minutes

Servings: 4

Ingredients:

- ½ pound of cold, fresh zucchini, sliced in half moons
- ½ pound of cold, fresh yellow squash, sliced in half moons
- ¼ pound of cold red pepper, julienned in strips ¼-inch thick
- ¼ pound of cold carrots, cut in ¼-inch strips a few inches long
- ¼ pound of cold red onions, thinly sliced
- 1 cold, small corn cob, cut crosswise in 1" segments
- 3 tablespoons of cold butter or margarine
- 1 teaspoon of salt
- 1 teaspoon of sugar
- ½ teaspoon of granulated garlic

- 1 teaspoon of Worcestershire sauce
- 1 teaspoon of soy sauce
- 2 teaspoons of fresh or dried parsley

Directions:

1. Wash, peel, and cut your vegetables as appropriate.
2. In a saucepan, heat the butter over medium-high heat.
3. Once it is hot, add it the salt, sugar, and garlic.
4. Add the carrots, squash, and zucchini, and when they start to soften add the rest of the vegetables and cook for a couple of minutes.
5. Add the Worcestershire sauce, soy sauce and parsley.
6. Stir to combine and coat the vegetables.
7. When all the vegetables are cooked to your preference, serve.

Nutrition: Calories: 170; Fat: 2g; Carbs: 18g; Protein: 15g

PF Chang's® Shanghai Cucumbers

Preparation Time: 5 Minutes

Cooking Time: 0 Minutes

Servings: 4

Ingredients:

- 2 English cucumbers, peeled and chopped
- 3 tablespoons of soy sauce
- ½ teaspoon of sesame oil
- 1 teaspoon of white vinegar
- Sprinkle of toasted sesame seeds

Directions:

1. Stir the soy sauce, sesame oil and vinegar in a serving dish.
2. Add the cucumbers and toss to coat.
3. Sprinkle with the sesame seeds.

Nutrition: Calories: 70; Fat: 3g; Carbs: 7g; Protein: 4g

Chili® Black Bean

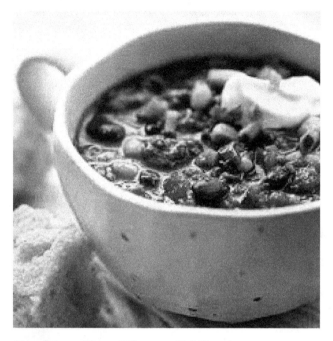

Preparation Time: 5 Minutes

Cooking Time: 25 Minutes

Servings: 6

Ingredients:

- 2 cans (15.5 ounces each) of black beans
- ½ teaspoon of sugar
- 1 teaspoon of ground cumin
- 1 teaspoon of chili powder
- ½ teaspoon of garlic powder
- 2 tablespoons of red onion, diced finely
- ½ teaspoon of fresh cilantro, minced (optional)
- ½ cup of water

- Salt and black pepper to taste
- Pico de Gallo and or sour cream for garnish (optional)

Directions:

1. Combine the beans, sugar, cumin, chili powder, garlic, onion, cilantro (if using), and water in a saucepan and mix well.
2. Over medium-low heat, let the bean mixture simmer for about 20-25 minutes. Season with salt and pepper to taste.
3. Remove the beans from heat and transfer to serving bowls.
4. Garnish with Pico de Gallo and a dollop of sour cream, if desired.

Nutrition: Calories: 143.8; Fat: 0.7g; Carbs: 25.9g; Protein: 9.5.2g

In "N" Out® Animal Style Fries

Preparation Time: 10 Minutes

Cooking Time: 30 Minutes

Servings: 6 to 8

Ingredients:

- 32 ounces of frozen French fries
- 2 cups of cheddar cheese, shredded
- 1 large onion, diced
- 2 tablespoons of raw sugar
- 2 tablespoons of olive oil
- 1 ½ cups of mayonnaise
- ¾ cup of ketchup
- ¼ cup of sweet relish
- 1 ½ teaspoons of white sugar
- 1 ½ teaspoons of apple cider vinegar
- ½ teaspoon of salt
- ½ teaspoon of black pepper

Directions:

1. Preheat oven to 350°F
2. Place the oven grill in the middle position.
3. Place fries on a large baking sheet and bake in the oven according to package's directions.
4. In the time being, warm the olive oil in a large non-stick skillet over medium heat.

5. Add the onions and sauté for about 2 minutes until fragrant and soft.

6. Add raw sugar and continue cooking until the onions caramelize.

7. Remove from heat and set aside.

8. Add the mayonnaise, ketchup, relish, white sugar, salt, and black pepper to a bowl and mix until well combined. Set aside.

9. Once the fries are cooked, remove from heat and set the oven to broil.

10. Sprinkle with the cheddar cheese over the fries and place under the broiler until the cheese melts, about 2–3 minutes.

11. Add the cheese fries to serving bowls or plates.

12. Add some caramelized onions on top and smother with mayonnaise sauce.

13. Serve immediately.

Nutrition: Calories: 750; Fat: 42g; Carbs: 54g; Protein: 19g

KFC® Coleslaw

Preparation Time: 15 Minutes

Cooking Time: 0 Minutes

Servings: 10

Ingredients:

- 8 cups of cabbage, finely diced
- ¼ cup of carrot, finely diced
- 2 tablespoons of onions, minced
- 1/3 cup of granulated sugar
- ½ teaspoon of salt
- 1/8 teaspoon of pepper
- ¼ cup of milk
- ½ cup of mayonnaise
- ¼ cup of buttermilk
- 1½ tablespoons of white vinegar
- 2½ tablespoons of lemon juice

Directions:

1. Mix the carrot, cabbage, and onions in a bowl.
2. Place the rest of the ingredients in a blender or food processor and blend until smooth.
3. Pour the sauce over the cabbage mixture.
4. Place in the fridge for more than a few hours before serving.

Nutrition: Calories: 170; Fat: 12g; Carbs: 14g; Protein: 4g

Cracker Barrel® Baby Carrot

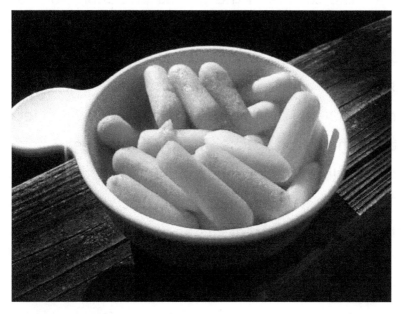

Preparation Time: 5 Minutes

Cooking Time: 45 Minutes

Servings: 6

Ingredients:

- 1 teaspoon of bacon grease, melted
- 2 pounds of fresh baby carrots
- Some water
- 1 teaspoon of salt
- ¼ cup of brown sugar
- ¼ cup of butter, melted
- ¼ cup of honey

Directions:

1. Heat the bacon grease in a pot.
2. Place the carrots in the grease and sauté for 10 seconds.
3. Cover the carrots with water and add the salt.
4. Bring the whole combination to a boil over medium heat, then reduce the heat to low and let it to simmer for another 30 to 45 minutes.
5. By this time, the carrots should be half cooked.
6. Take away half the water from the pot and add the rest of the ingredients.
7. Keep cooking until the carrots become tender.
8. Transfer to a bowl and serve.

Nutrition: Calories: 80, Fat: 1g, Carbs: 18g, Protein: 1g

Olive Garden Gnocchi with Spicy Tomato and Wine Sauce

Preparation Time: 10 Minutes

Cooking Time: 40 Minutes

Servings: 4

Ingredients:

Sauce:

- 2 tablespoons of extra virgin olive oil
- 6 fresh garlic cloves
- ½ teaspoon of chili flakes
- 1 cup of dry white wine
- 1 cup of chicken broth
- 2 cans (14.5 ounces each) of tomatoes
- ¼ cup of fresh basil, chopped
- ¼ cup of sweet creamy butter, cut into 1-inch cubes, chilled
- ½ cup of parmesan cheese, freshly grated

Pasta:

- 1 pound of gnocchi
- Salt, to taste
- Black pepper, freshly crushed, to taste

Directions:

1. Place the garlic, olive oil, and chili flakes in a cold pan and cook over medium heat.
2. Once the garlic starts turning golden brown, add the wine and broth and bring the mixture to a simmer.
3. After about 10 minutes, the broth should be halved.
4. When that happens, add in the tomatoes and basil and then let the sauce continue simmering for another 30 minutes.
5. When the sauce has condensed, set it aside to cool for 3 minutes.
6. After 3 minutes, place the sauce in a blender, and add the butter and parmesan.
7. Purée everything together and set aside.
8. Prepare the pasta by boiling the gnocchi in a large pot.
9. When it is cooked, strain the pasta and mix with the sauce.
10. Transfer everything to a plate and serve.

Nutrition: Calories: 285.8; Fat: 18.9g; Carbs: 12.1g; Protein: 8.4g;
Sodium: 476.9mg

Chipotle® Sofritas

Preparation Time: 10 Minutes

Cooking Time: 25 Minutes

Servings: 4

Ingredients:

Mexican Spice Mix:

- ½ teaspoon of dried oregano leaves
- 2 teaspoons of ancho chili powder, ground
- 1 teaspoon of cumin, ground
- ½ teaspoon of coriander, ground
- ½ teaspoon of kosher salt

Sofritas:

- 1 tablespoon of avocado or olive oil
- ½ medium onion, diced
- 2 garlic cloves, minced
- 1 teaspoon of chipotle chili in adobo sauce, minced
- 1 tablespoon of mild Hatch chili, diced
- 1 tablespoon of Mexican Spice Mix
- 2 tablespoons of tomato paste
- 1 package (16 ounces) of organic extra firm tofu, drained, dried, crumbled
- 1 cup of your favorite Mexican beer
- Salt and black pepper to taste

- Tortillas and lime wedges for garnish

Directions:

1. Place all the Mexican Spice Mix ingredients in a container or plastic bag and shake to mix.
2. Sauté the onion and garlic in oil over medium heat for 5 minutes.
3. Mix in both the chilies and the spice mix and sauté for another minute.
4. Pour in the tomato paste and cook for a minute.
5. Add the rest of the ingredients and cook for 5 more minutes.
6. Taste and regulate seasoning with salt and pepper if required.
7. Remove the mixture from heat, transfer to a bowl, and then serve with tortillas and thin lime wedges.

Nutrition: Calories: 470, Fat: 19g, Carbs: 59g, Protein: 16g, Sodium: 1160mg

Melting Pot® Green Goddess Dip

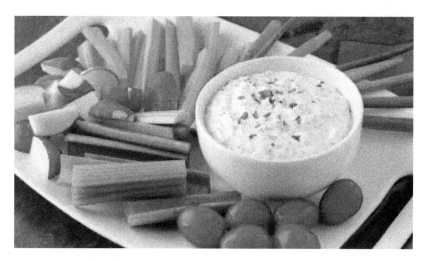

Preparation Time: 5 Minutes

Cooking Time: 5 Minutes

Servings: 12

Ingredients:

- 8 ounces of cheese, sliced
- 1/2 cup of milk
- 1/4 cup of cream
- 2 tbsp. of onion
- 2 tbsp. of parsley
- 2 tbsp. of chives

Directions:

1. Microwave cheese and milk in a healthy container for 2–4 minutes, whisking after each minute,

before adding the cream cheese. Melt and mix smoothly.

2. Stir in sour cream, cabbage, chives, and parsley.
3. Refrigerate before serving and enjoy!

Nutrition: Calories: 85, Fat: 7.8g, Carbs: 1.6g, Protein: 1.6g

Applebee's Onion Peels

Preparation Time: 5 Minutes

Cooking Time: 25 Minutes

Servings: 4 to 6

Ingredients:

Horseradish dipping sauce:

- 1/2 cup of mayonnaise
- 1 tbsp. of prepared horseradish
- 2 tsp. of white vinegar
- 1 tsp. of water
- 1 tsp. of paprika
- 1 tsp. of ketchup
- 1/4 tsp. of black pepper
- 1/8 tsp. of dried oregano
- 1/8 tsp. of cayenne
- 1/4 tsp. of garlic powder
- 1/4 tsp. of onion powder

Batter:

- 5–6 cups of shortening
- 1 large onion
- 1/2 cup of all-purpose flour
- 1/2 cup of Progresso Plain Bread Crumbs
- 1/2 tsp. of salt
- 1/2 tsp. of black pepper

- 1 1/2 cups of milk

Directions:

1. Make horseradish dipping sauce, mixing ingredients with a whisk in a medium cup.
2. Then blend the sauce until smooth, cover, and chill.
3. Heat the shortening on a deep fryer to 350°F.
4. Slice the end of the stem and the end of the root off the onion, then cut through the onion, slice it in half with the onion lying on a flat side. Slice each half 4 to 5 times more to make onion wedges in a spoken fashion.
5. Separate pieces of an onion.
6. Mix all the dry fixings into a medium bowl to make batter.
7. Whisk in the milk until smooth batter then let the batter sit for 5 minutes. It should grow thicker.
8. Then again whisk the batter.
9. Dip pieces of onion in the batter, when the oil is hot, let some of the batter drip off, and then cautiously drop the piece of coated onion into the hot oil.
10. Repeat for 1 to 2 minutes, or until light brown, frying 8 to 12 at a time.
11. Drain onto a towel rack or notebook.

12. Repeat until the onion is removed, stack the newer lots on top of the old lots to keep them dry.

13. Serve fried onion slices on a plate or in a paper-coated basket with horseradish dipping sauce on the side when they are all done.

Nutrition: Calories: 234, Fat: 14g, Carbs: 22g, Protein: 5g

DESSERT RECIPES

Lime Pie

Preparation Time: 20 minutes

Cooking Time: 20 minutes

Servings: 8

Ingredients:

Crust

- ½ cup almond flour
- ½ cup coconut flour sifted
- ¼ cup granulated Erythritol
- ¼ cup unsalted butter, melted
- 2 organic eggs
- ¼ teaspoon salt

Filling

- ¾ cup unsweetened coconut milk
- ½ cup granulated Erythritol
- ¼ cup heavy cream
- 2 teaspoons xanthan gum
- 1 teaspoon guar gum
- ¼ teaspoon powdered stevia
- 3 organic egg yolks

- ½ cup fresh key lime juice
- 2 tablespoons unsweetened dried coconut

Topping

- 1 cup whipped cream
- ½ key lime, cut into slices

Directions:

1. Preheat your oven to 4000F.
2. For the crust:
3. Add all ingredients in a bowl and mix until well combined.
4. With your hands, knead the dough for about 1 minute.
5. Make a ball from the dough.
6. Arrange the dough ball between 2 sheets of wax paper and with a rolling pin, roll into a 1/8-inch-thick circle.
7. In a 9-inch pie dish, place the dough and with your hands, press the mixture in the bottom and upsides.
8. Now, with a fork, prick the bottom and sides of crust at many places.
9. Bake for approximately 10 minutes.
10. Remove from the oven and place the crust onto a wire rack to cool.

11.   Now, set the temperature of the oven to 3500F (1800C).

For filling:

1. In a food processor, add the coconut milk, Erythritol, heavy cream, xanthan gum, guar gum, and stevia, and pulse until well combined.
2. Add the egg yolks and lime juice and pulse until well combined.
3. Place the filling mixture over the crust and with the back of a spoon spread evenly.
4. Bake for approximately 10 minutes.
5. Remove from the oven and place the pie dish onto a wire rack to cool for about 10 minutes.
6. Now, freeze the pie for about 3−4 hours before serving.
7. Remove from the freezer and garnish the pie with the whipped cream and lemon slices.
8. Cut into desired-sized slices and serve.

Nutrition: 251 Calories 24g Fat 5g Protein

Peanut Butter Fudge

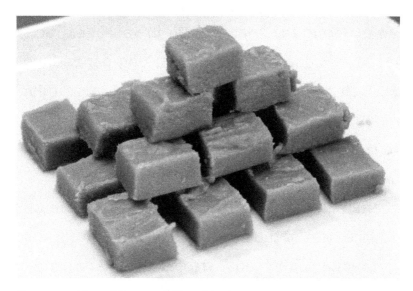

Preparation Time: 10 minutes

Cooking Time: 5 minutes

Servings: 16

Ingredients:

- 1½ cups creamy, salted peanut butter
- 1/3 cup butter
- 2/3 cup powdered Erythritol
- ¼ cup unsweetened Protein powder
- 1 teaspoon organic vanilla extract

Directions:

1. First, in a small pan, add peanut butter and butter over low heat and cook until melted and smooth.

2. Add the Erythritol and Protein powder and mix until smooth.

3. Remove from the heat and stir in vanilla extract.

4. Place the fudge mixture onto baking paper-lined 8x8-inch baking dish evenly and with a spatula, smooth the top surface.

5. Freeze for about 30–45 minutes or until set completely.

6. Carefully transfer the fudge onto a cutting board with the help of the parchment paper.

7. Cut the fudge into equal-sized squares and serve.

Nutrition: 184 Calories 16g Fat 7g Protein

Mascarpone Brownies

Preparation Time: 15 minutes

Cooking Time: 28 minutes

Servings: 16

Ingredients:

- 5 ounces unsweetened dark chocolate, chopped roughly
- 4 tablespoons unsalted butter
- 3 large organic eggs
- ½ cup Erythritol
- ¼ cup mascarpone cheese
- ¼ cup cacao powder, divided
- ½ teaspoon salt

Directions:

1. Preheat the oven to 3750F.
2. Line a 9x9-inch baking sheet with a parchment paper.
3. In a medium microwave-safe bowl, add the chocolate and microwave on High for about 2 minutes or until melted completely, stirring after every 30 seconds.
4. Add the butter and microwave for about 1 minute or until melted and smooth, stirring once every 10 seconds.

5. Now, remove from the microwave and stir until smooth.

6. Set aside to cool slightly.

7. In a large bowl, add the eggs and Erythritol and with an electric mixer, beat on high speed until frothy.

8. And then, add the mascarpone cheese and beat until smooth.

9. Add 2 tablespoons of the cacao powder and salt and gently stir to combine.

10. Now, sift in the remaining cacao powder and stir until well combined.

11. Add the melted chocolate mixture into the egg mixture and mix well until well combined.

12. Place the mixture into the prepared pan evenly.

13. Bake for approximately 25 minutes.

14. Remove from the oven and let it cool completely before cutting.

15. With a sharp knife, cut into desired sized squares and serve.

Nutrition: 93 Calories 9g Fat 3g Protein

Keto Brownies

Preparation Time: 30 minutes

Cooking Time: 0 minutes

Servings: 12

Ingredients:

- 6 ounces coconut oil; melted
- 4 ounces cream cheese
- 5 tablespoons swerve sweetener
- 6 eggs
- 2 teaspoons vanilla
- 3 ounces of cocoa powder
- 1/2 teaspoon baking powder

Directions:

1. In the blender, mix eggs with coconut oil, cocoa powder, baking powder, vanilla, cream cheese, and swerve. Stir using the mixer.
2. Pour this into the lined baking dish, introduce in the oven at 350 degrees F and bake for 20 minutes
3. Slice into rectangle pieces when it gets cold and serve

Nutrition: 184 Calories 17g Fat 1.4g Protein

Raspberry and Coconut

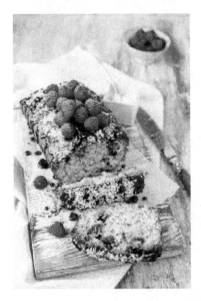

Preparation Time: 15 minutes

Cooking Time: 0 minutes

Servings: 12

Ingredients:

- 1/4 cup swerve sweetener
- 1/2 cup coconut oil
- 1/2 cup raspberries; dried
- 1/2 cup coconut; shredded
- 1/2 cup coconut butter

Directions:

1. In your food processor, blend dried berries very well.
2. Heat the pan with the butter over medium heat.

3. Add oil, coconut and swerve; stir and cook for 5 minutes

4. Pour half of this into the lined baking pan and spread well.

5. Add raspberry powder and also spread.

6. Top with the rest of the butter mix spread and keep in the fridge

7. Cut into pieces and serve

Nutrition: 401 Calories 42g Fat 8g Protein

CONCLUSION

Hopefully, these recipes have given you a few tips and tricks on how to recreate your favorite restaurant dishes at home.

The book is meant to give you some motivation and inspiration to cook these meals in the comforts of your own home. No need to dine out to satisfy your cravings for these popular dishes. At least this way you will know exactly what your food went through before arriving at your plate and will save a few bucks in the process. And maybe the next time you decide to dine out, you'll dine in instead

Always remember when doing copycat recipes. The first thing you must do is look at the recipe itself. If it's not posted, don't even think about doing it. Some restaurants have contracts with companies that protect their recipes and if you have a copy without permission, you could be getting sued.

Next, read the directions and the ingredients list to see if there are any substitutions that must be made or if the number of servings has changed. If you are able to locate the recipe, it's time to start gathering your ingredients. Print out a copy and go grocery shopping.

It takes a lot of work to make a restaurant copycat recipe. There are many parts that go into making a successful dish at home, and it is important not to skip any steps. When all the prep work is done, it's time to start cooking. Use a deep pot for boiling and a sauté pan for searing or frying. Turn on the burner and let the pan get hot before adding oil or butter.

After you've got your ingredients simmering or sautéing away, it's time to add in any extra toppings, such as cheese or sour cream. Once the dish is done, you can add in seasonings or garnishes to give it a restaurant-quality presentation. Finally, serve up your meal and enjoy it!

First of all, I want to thank you for buying our book, which was the result of a long period of work for us.

We always try to give my best in our books to offer the reader the highest possible experience. All contents are enriched and analyzed in detail so that you can find the solutions you were looking for in our manuscripts.

We hope we have responded, even if in part, to your expectations.

We will be grateful if you could leave your own review on Amazon. This would be really important to us and our work. We promise that we will read your opinion with interest.

9 781801 830478